Marijuana Strains That Promote Sexual Arousal

I0413990

And How To Grow Them

by Michael Blood, M.S.W.

Note to the reader:

These strains are presented in the following order:

Those with the strongest reports of sexual arousal are pushed toward the top of the list. Those with the greatest frequency of reported negative side effects are pushed toward the bottom. The result is that the first 30 or 35 strains at the top tend to have very minimal or no negative side effects reported and tend to be the highest in reports of sexual arousal.

Negative side effects are considered to be the following: Headaches, Dizziness, Paranoia and Anxiety. (not considered "negative" side effects are Dry Eyes and Dry Mouth which are both common in most strains).

That being said, it should always be remembered that cannabis is an herb who's effects are subjective to the individual and the environment.

Lastly, all information herein is based on subjective reports of individuals and not upon "scientific, double-blind testing."

This book further assumes all use of marijuana will take place exclusively in states where use is legal. The Author is not prescribing nor claiming the effectiveness of the strains reported here, but simply passing on information reported in the literature, on-line and by word of mouth. Again, all subjective data. Anyone suffering E.D. or other sexual disorders should consult an M.D.

Table of Contents:

Canna Sutra 70/30 indica dom cross 13 to 17%THC (Reclining Buddha x Sensi Star) by Delta 9 Labs Tastes like sweet incense with a hashy flavor. Designed for indoor growing but does fine outdoors in Mediterranean climates. Flowers for 9 to 10 weeks. Yield indoors is 300 to 500g /m² likes feeding but not overwatering. Does best when given plenty of root space and space to develop
multiple branches. Responds well to super-cropping. Buds are airy until the last week when they harden.
Good For: Mood, Sexual Arousal, Depression, Insomnia, Pain, Stress, Clarity, Asthma
Possible Side Effects: Will make you "pitch a tent" Should be used with someone with whom you want to be intimate. Dry Mouth is the side effect reported. NOTE lack of reported negative side effects.

Sexxpot indica dominant cross   14%THC
(Mr. Nice x Unknown) by Karyn Wagne. Bred by a woman specifically to facilitate female orgasm: depth of pleasure, duration and ease of attainment. No additional information is available.
Good For: Sexual Arousal, Pain, Stress, Relaxation
Possible Side Effects: Not listed

Stitch's Love Potion 80/20 sativa dom cross 17%THC AUTOFLOWERING Grows indoors/outdoors 2 to 3.5 ft. 73 days from seed to harvest. Yields 40 to 110g/plant
Good For: Erotic Arousal, Depression
Possible Side Effects: Uplifting, feel great, Reputation for Sexual arousal is strong.

CBD Critical Cure (aka **Critical Cure) 80/20 indica dom cross (Critical Kush **x** ruderalis) 8%CBD and 5%THC Smells like sweet earth with spicy lemon. Taste is mild sweet peppery citrus with lemoney earth. Grows well indoors or greenhouses. Plants are 20 to 40 inches. Flowers for 7 to 8.5 weeks. Yield is 600+g/m²
Good   For: Sexual   Arousal,   Pain,   Stress, Inflammation,   Nausea,
Possible Side Effects: Happy, Dizziness, Headache, Dry Mouth, Dry Eyes

The Flav 60/40 indica dominant cross 13 to 19%THC (Romulan x Space Queen) One of *High Times'* "Top 10" in 2008Taste is said to be amazing. Balanced indica - sativa effects. Flowers for 7 to 8.5 weeks indoors or out. Yield is "high."
Good For: Sexual Arousal, Stress, Appetite, Nausea
Possible Side Effects: Relaxed, Euphoric, Dry Mouth, Dry Eyes. A very small minority of patients reported Dizziness, Anxiety and/or Headache.

Thor's Hammer 90/10 sativa dom cross 21%THC
(Vortex x Cinerella 99 x Acapulco Gold)
Name Ref: Hits you hard, like Thor's hammer. Grows
well indoors or out with exceptionally huge, sticky colas.
Referred to as, "A cultivator's dream." Another source
called it, "a workhorse" and it is said to be excellent for
cross breading, retaining its form and integrating
positive qualities of the strain with which it is crossed.
Flowering time is very short for a sativa: 9 to 10 weeks.
Yield is "Large"
Good For: Sexual Arousal, Stress, Inflammation,
Creativity, Energy
Possible Side Effects: Euphoria, Dry Mouth, a very
small portion of patients reported Dry Eyes and/or
Paranoia.

Tommy's Home Grown   19%THC
(AKA **THG**) 50/50 cross (named after Tommy Chong
of Cheech & Chong) Handled exclusively by Encanto
Green Cross Medical Marijuana Dispensary in Phoenix,
AZ with no growing information available.
Good For: Stress, Sexual Arousal, Appetite, Focus
Possible Side Effects: Energetic, Relaxed, Happy.
        NOTE: No negative side effects reported.

Thaidal Wave sativa dominant cross   %THC Unk.
but powerful (Thai Landrace x Skunk) Unknown
breeder. Originated in Thailand. No horticultural
information available.

Good For: Anxiety, Stress, Energy, Migraine, Creativity, Sexual Arousal
Possible Side Effects: hits like a big wave. Euphoric, super-focused, feel very content & right with the world. Potency not reported. Few experience Dizziness.

Hawaiian Diesel 100% sativa cross   22%THC
(Hawaiian land race x Diesel) Pure sativa which grows best indoors but should do well outdoors in a Mediterranean or tropical climate. Aroma of fresh citrus and pine. Tastes like sweet tropical fruit. Considered one of the finest strains by many. Seeds or cuttings ("clones") are best grown indoors in most climates, in a hydroponic setup. Flowers 8 to 10 weeks. Yield unreported.
Good For: Stress, Sexual Arousal, Relaxation, Socializing, Energetic, Giggles
Possible Side Effects: Dry Mouth, minority reported Dry Eyes. NOTE lack of reported negative side effects.

Buffalo Bill 70/30 sativa dom cross   25 to 28%THC
(Willie's Wonder x Killer Chemdog) by New House Seeds Some say the second parent is Killer Ken, others Killer Chem, but New House Seeds says it is Killer Chemdog. Spicy fruity smell. Taste is spicy lemon. No grow information available at time of publication.
Good For: Fatigue, Sexual Arousal, Relaxation, Cramps, Muscle Spasms
Possible Side Effects: Euphoria, Dry Mouth. Super

Strong. NOTE lack of reported negative side effects

Black Label Kush indica   8 to23%THC
(Afghani indica land strain 1 x Afghani indica land

strain 2) One of the lesser known indicas, it has a
strongly pungent smell and strong medical effects.
Flowers for 7 to 8 weeks. Yield is 400 to 500g/m²
It is highly valued by those who can find it.
Good For: Anxiety, Insomnia, Relaxation, Stress,
Pain, Eye Pressure, Sexual Arousal, Migraines
Possible Side Effects: Negative side effects are quite
minimal, and include Dry Eyes, but very few
reports of Dry Mouth, and almost no Dizziness.
Paranoia even less. Excellent choice for beginner
patients with above symptoms.

Doug's Varin sativa cross high THCV 22 to 24%THC
(selective phenotypes of Harlequin repeatedly selected
and crossed back for several generations) by Dougie's
Farm near Sacramento, CA. Very new and nearly
impossible to get at time of publication, though
Elemental Wellness in San Jose, CA was provided
with 3 plants and they MAY have some available.
Smells of earthy pine and sweet citrus. A rare sativa
strain that was specially crafted to contain high
amounts of the cannabinoid THCV, a psychoactive
cannabis compound known to be effective treating:
Good For: Panic Attacks, Parkinson's, Tremors,

Stimulate Bone Growth, Energy, Suppression of
Appetite, Sexual Arousal, Creativity, Energy, Focus,
Inflammation, Nausea, Stress, PTSD, Parkinson's
Disease, Chronic Pain. Motivation, Tinnitus
Possible Side Effects: Patient's suffering from
anorexia and appetite loss should steer clear of Doug's

Varin, as THCV suppresses hunger. Immediate focus,
motivation and creative without feeling overwhelmed.
Effects of this strain are relatively short lived.

Sour Chunk 80/20 sativa dom cross   12% THC
(Deep Chunk x East Coast Sour Diesel). Other
sources list at an indica dominant strain. The plants
look indica like but medicates like a sativa. Grows well
in all mediums and responds especially well to SCROG
set up. Flowers for10 weeks Yield: No reports.
NOTE: This is a "clone only" strain.
Good For: Stress, Relaxation, Cramps, Headaches,
Insomnia, Pain, Sexual Arousal
Possible Side Effects: Daytime med. Euphoric, Happy,
Dry Eyes, few reported Anxiety, Dizziness, Dry Mouth.

Island Sweet Skunk sativa dom cross   %THC Unk.
levels, but people rank it 10 out of 10 for potency.
Requires staking to support exceptionally large buds,
Indoors/out, yields are "insanely high" SOG indoors
results in no vegetation time. Odor when growing is
"strongest" of all strains. Flowers for 9 to 11 weeks.
Good For: Nausea, Appetite, Focus, ADD/ADHD,

Pain, Sexual Arousal

Possible Side Effects: daytime smoke, energetic, ability to focus is greatly increased, enjoyable. Colors more vibrant, music is enhanced, forget about any pain.
Said to be a very powerful sexual stimulant; increasing sensation, stamina, and libido quite dramatically.
Potency: very powerful. 1 hit recommended, 2 Max.

Dr. Funk (AKA **Dr. Funkenstein**)

80/20 indica dom cross $THC Unk.
(Bluberry x Bubba Kush) by unknown breeder
NOTE: some are selling a strain of this name that is actually DJ Short Blueberry x Bubba Kush – another listing has it as Tahoe OG X Ken's OG. There are indications of other crosses being referred to as Dr. Funk. Comments here refer to the strain from the first listed parents. Tastes like sweet berry and has an earthy taste on the exhale. In addition to the dubiously named strains, to make matters worse, no grow information can be found. If you want this strain, you must be sure of what cross you are getting.
Good For: Sexual Arousal, Pain, Stress, Insomnia, Depression, Headaches.
Possible Side Effects: Happiness, Euphoria, Dry Mouth NOTE: No negative side effects reported.

Purple Sage 65/35 sativa dom cross   16%THC
(SAGE x Unk. purple mix) Exceptionally easy to grow, tolerant of pests and uneven nutrients.
Pleasing aroma during growth. May be prone to

hermaphroditing. No other growing information available.
Good For: Sexual Arousal, Creativity, Stress, Fatigue and Pain.
Possible Side Effects: Dry Mouth, Dry Eyes.
NOTE lack of reported negative side effects.

BC Big Bud 65/35 sativa dom cross 12 to 16%THC (Big Bud x Unk. sativa strains) sativa parents vary among breeders. Smells like an earthy skunk. Tastes like earthy sweet berries. Indoors SOG or SCROG setup is best. Outdoors it will require netting or other support for its HUGE buds. Flowers 8 to 8.5 weeks. Yield HUGE
Good For: Sexual Arousal, Stress, Pain, Nausea, Eye Pressure, Appetite, Relaxation, Insomnia, Depression.
Possible Side Effects: Extreme Euphoria, Dry Mouth, some Dry Eyes. About 15% of patients report Anxiety, and/or Paranoia and/or Dizziness.

Sweet Kush 50/50 cross   18%THC (Sweet Tooth x OG Kush) Another source: says (Kush x South African Sativa) Can grow to 10 feet outdoors, but also does well indoors. Covered in trichomes and said to make terrific hash, even from leaves. Plants produce tight, compact colas. Flowers 7 to 8 weeks. Yield to 500g/m² indoors and more outdoors.
Good For: Pain, Stress, Headaches, Insomnia, Muscle Spasms, Sexual Arousal, Giggles
Possible Side Effects: Relaxed, Euphoric, Dry Mouth, Dry Eyes, some reported Paranoia, Dizziness, Headache

Jack Frost cross   16 to 23%THC
Jack Herrer x White Widow x Northern Lights #5
x Rainbow Kashmiri) by Goldenseed Tastes like
earthy/woody/piney. Jack Frost is said to have
the highest concentration of trichomes which makes

it the easiest strain from which to make kief. Likes
SOG setup. Indoors/out grow. Flowers for 8 weeks.
Yield is "good"   Do not top this plant.
Good For: Social events, Writing, Anxiety, Sexual
Arousal, Stress, Appetite, Brainstorming, Depression,
Fatigue
Possible Side Effects: Will promote doing chores,
multi-tasking. Very Uplifting. Prolongs Sexual Arousal,
Potency: moderate. Dry Mouth, some reported Dry
Eyes, Anxiety, Paranoia and/or Dizziness.

Chucky's Bride sativa dominant cross up to 20%THC
Exodus Chese x Cinderella 99) by Eskobar Seeds
Smell is complex mixture of sweet citrus, pineapple,
pungent, skunky cheese. Taste is similar to smell with a
chemical cheesy twist. Some users find
the taste off putting. Good grower indoors/outdoors
or greenhouse. Flowers 7 to 8 weeks. Yield 500g/m^2
Good For: Tinnitus, Depression, Pain, Giggles,
Mood, Sexual Arousal, Creativity
Possible Side Effects: Euphoria, Dry Mouth,
NOTE lack of reported negative side effects.

Love Potion #9 60/40 indica dom cross   to 26%THC
(Northern Lights #5 x Love Potion #5) exceptionally tasty
increasing as one smokes. Further info unavailable
Good For: Giggles, Relaxation, Creativity, Inflammation,
Depression, Stress, Pain, Anxiety, Stress, Night Terrors,

Sexual Arousal.
Possible Side Effects: Instant "stone" Initially Couch
Lock then Euphoria. Headache, very little Dry Mouth
reported almost no Dizziness. Exceptionally powerful!

Wet Dream 90/10 sativa dom cross   15 to 22%THC
(Blue Dream x Ocean Beach Haze) Another strain from
San Diego – the Ocean Beach area. While specific
growing information is not available it does well indoors,
SCROG, and outdoors can become HUGE. Has small to
medium-sized buds - an easy grow for the beginner.
Good For: Sexual Arousal, Creativity, Stress, Migraines
Possible Side Effects: Immediate, Energetic, Euphoria,
Dry Mouth, few report Dizziness, Dry Eyes and very few
reported Headache.

Ms. Universe sativa dominant cross   14 to 20%THC
(Des*tar x Space Queen) by Dynasty Seeds
4 phenotypes denoted primarily based on their
Taste & Smell: 1)Pineapple (40%), 2)Berry (30%),
3)Tallest, variety of smells (10%), 4)Haze (20%),
Flowering time varies somewhat with phenotype,
about 9 to 10 weeks. Yield to 550g /m^2

Good For: Erotic Arousal, Pain, Stress, Giggles
Possible Side Effects: ONE hit, Psychedelic,
Dry Mouth, Relaxed, Happy, Euphoric.
NOTE lack of negative side effects reported.

Opal OG Kush

80/20 indica dominant cross   15 to 26%THC
(Frankenstein x Lemon OG Kush) by Nine Point
Industries Growth. It grows best indoors in soil.
Flowering time 8 to 9 weeks. Easy grow, Yields 475g/m²
Good For: Stress, Nausea, Insomnia, Headache, Sexual
Arousal
Possible Side Effects: Immediate effects, Euphoria,
Red Eyes, Dry Mouth. Very few reported Dizziness
and/or Paranoia

Grape Drink (NOT Grape Drunk)

70/30 indica dom cross to 19%THC
(Kibo Kush x Grape God) Sweet smell with a candy
sweet taste. New strain with no horticultural
information provided yet.
Good For: Creativity, Giggles, Stress, Pain, Depression
Sexual Arousal
Possible Side Effects: Happy, talkative. If smoked a
lot, sleep results. No negative side effects yet reported.

OG Wreck (AKA Wreck OG)

70/30 sativa dom cross   15 to 18%THC
(OG Kush x Trainwreck) Zero information available re yield, flowering time, etc
Good For: Sexual Arousal, Nausea, Appetite, Fatigue, Depression, Headaches, Stress
Possible Side Effects: Couchlock, Euphoric, Dry Eyes, Dry Mouth, a minority reported Anxiety and/or Paranoia

Kushage 60/40   sativa dominant cross   18%THC
(OG Kush x SAGE) Tastes of hints of pine and citrus, Flowers for 10 to 11 weeks, lots of branches. Yield to over 400g /m²
Good For: Sexual Arousal, Energetic & Creative, Pain
Possible Side Effects: effects come on very softly. Regardless of age, it makes one feel like a young Lover. Euphoria, Dry Eyes, Dry Mouth, few reported Dizziness, fewer Paranoia, fewer still reported Headache.

Guava Chem sativa dominant cross   to 21%THC
(Tres Chemdawg x Chem #4) Tastes like citrus, guava and papaya. It has a sweet aroma. Flowering time is 7 weeks. No info on yield is available, but buds are described as "great" from which one might infer "large," which would, therefore, imply at good yield.
Good For: Sexual Arousal, Depression, Pain, Muscle Spasms, Stress, Inflammation, Anxiety, Giggles, Creativity
Possible Side Effects: Happy, Euphoric, Dry Eyes, Few reported Dry Mouth, Paranoia and almost no reports of Anxiety and/or Dizziness.

LA Confidential indica   20 to 24%THC

(Afghani Land Race x OG LA Affie) by DNA Genetics
4 ft indoors, much taller outdoors. Taste is described
as "piney" and the smell as skunky. 2006 High Times
Strain of the Year as well as numerous Cannabis Cups
throughout several years. Smells like dank, woody

spices, tastes like butternut squash with nutmeg.
Flowers 7 to 8 weeks, Yield is 300 to 500g/m2,
Good For: PTSD, Stress. Pain, Insomnia, Nausea,
Appetite, Sex, Bi-polar Disorder, Autism
Possible Side Effects: Euphoria along with uplifting
(unusual for an Indica) Dry Mouth, some report Dry
Eyes, few report Dizziness, Paranoia and/or Headache.

Northern Lights #5

95/5 indica dom cross   22 to 26%THC
Won 3 Cannabis Cups No other information available.
Good For: Sexual Arousal, Hypertension, Muscle
Spasms, Depression, Stress, Anxiety, Apatite, Creativity,
Spinal Cord Injury
Possible Side Effects: functional "high." Very clear,
euphoric, creative thoughts. STRONG 5 to10 seconds
after exhale - lasts 3 to 4hrs. Dry Mouth, Dry Eyes, A
minority of patients reported Headache, Paranoia
and very few report Dizziness.

Himalayan Gold 60/40 indica dom cross   15%THC

(Nepal land strains x North Indian land strains)
5ft indoors, to 8 ft outdoors, easy grow. Flowers 8 to 9

weeks, yields 600 to 1,000g /m² – outdoors 1,500g/plant

Good For: Migraines, Pain, Creativity, Sexual Arousal, Insomnia

Possible Side Effects: Mild head high, daytime use, patients new to cannabis. Daytime mellow, Potency is

moderate. Dry Eyes, Dry Mouth, few reported Paranoia, very few Dizziness.

Caramella 80/20 indica dom cross   15 to 20%THC by Homegrown Fantaseeds. Smells like butterscotch caramel and Tastes like it, too. Considered one of the best tasting of all strains. Grows easily indoors or out, even for beginners. The plants are robust with long colas covered in sticky resin which also cove the entire plant. Does well in soil or hydroponics, likes SOG and in such cases should be planted 20/m² Flowering time is 8 to 9 weeks. Yield is described as "moderate."

Good For: Spasticity, Insomnia, Eye Pressure, Sexual Arousal, Pain, Relaxation, Socializing, Migraines, MS

Possible Side Effects: Dry Eyes, Euphoria. NOTE lack of reported negative side effects

Northern Wreck 70/30 indica dom cross   29%THC (Northern Lights x Train Wreck) Flowering time is 10 Yield is described as "very heavy."

Good For: Sexual Arousal, Pain, Stress, Insomnia, Depression

Possible Side Effects: Relaxed, Happy Dry Mouth, A tiny minority of patients report dizziness

Master Jedi 75/25 indica dominant cross to 25%THC (Skywalker x Master Kush) Indoor/outdoor grow. No further information, but check the parent strains as reasonable predictors.
Good For: Sexual Arousal, Stress, Depression, Giggles, Pain, Muscle Spasms
Possible Side Effects: Relaxation, Euphoria, Dry Mouth, Dry Eyes with a small minority of patients reporting Dizziness, Headache and/or Paranoia

Pink Kush 90/10 indica dominant cross 20%THC (MAY be a phenotype of OG Kush") Tastes like sweet vanilla candied perfume. Smells like pine wood and flowers. After flowering starts the plants can grow up to 75% taller. Flowers 10 to 11 weeks. Yield is "high."
Good For: Stress, Pain, Insomnia, Depression, Nausea
Possible Side Effects: Little required for medical results. Extremely strong. Intense euphoria common. Dry Mouth, Dry Eyes, very little Dizziness, even less Paranoia, almost no Anxiety reported.

Purple People Eater indica dom cross %THC Unk. ({Lapis Mnt. Indica x GDP} X {Afghan x Purple Urkle}) Purple buds, said to do as well cropped or with a SOG or SCROG setup. Yield is said to be "low-average" but the resulting buds are highly prized. No other info on

Yield or other growing aspects of this strain.
Good For: Sexual Arousal, Mood Lifter, Depression, Stress
Possible Side Effects: Uplifted, Relaxed. Others not given

Zensation 75/25 indica dom cross 20 to 24%THC by Minitry of Cannabis. Hydroponic grow or soil. Flowering 8 to 9 weeks. Yields 400g/plant outdoors.
Good For: Sexual Interest, Anxiety, Pain, Insomnia
Possible Side Effects:: Very Strong and Very long lasting. Promotes sexual interest, not specifically energy.

Bubblicious 70/30 indica dom cross 15 to 20% THC (Original Bubblegum x F1 Lavender) by Nirvana Seeds Smells like Bubblegum. Tastes like fruity Bubblegum. Grows well indoors/outdoors. Considered THE BEST due to smell, taste, medical efficiency and near zero negative side effects by many if not most patients that have used it. Plants are short. Flower for 8 to 11 weeks. Yield is 400 to 500g/m^2 in a SOG setup.
Good For: Sexual Arousal, Stress, Appetite, Depression, Insomnia, Relaxation, Pain
Possible Side Effects: Happy, Euphoric, Dry Mouth, some reported Dizziness and/or Dry Eyes. Excellent medication due to very low frequency of negative side effects.

Bhang Afgoo indica C02 extract 50-65% THC. Natural 25 to 35%THC Afgoo by Bhang is an indica strain that has been processed into a variety of oil-based products compatible with the Bhang Stick portable vaporizer.

Purple Pinecone indica dominant cross 10 to 19%THC by Sagarmatha Seeds. Intense smell pine and earth. Plants only about 2 ft. Excellent indoors and fine outdoors. Flowers for 7 to 8 weeks. Yield 350g /m^2 Highly regarded.
Good For: Sexual Arousal, Relaxation, Appetite, Mood, Insomnia
Possible Side Effects: Headache, Euphoric, Dry Eyes, Dry Mouth, Dizziness.

White Zombie 60/40 indica dom cross 15 to 19%THC Two theories exist as to the name – one is that it contains Zombie OG DNA, the other is that the breeder was a Rob Zombie fan. Buds are large, dense and have orange hairs. Further information on cultivation is not available.
Good For: Sexual Arousal, Stress, Pain, Depression Creativity and Anorexia
Possible Side Effects: Happy, Dry Eyes, Dry Mouth, Dizziness and a minority reported Paranoia

Gravity indica dom cross   high CBD content   20%THC

(Hash Plant x Northern Lights) Other strains of this same name are also known. Smells and tastes like sweet and sour fruit. Further information is not available on this strain.

Good For: Sexual Arousal, Pain, Stress, Fatigue

Possible Side Effects: Night time use, Happy, Euphoric, Dry Eyes, Dry Mouth, a minority of patients reported Dizziness, Headache and/or Paranoia

Wonder Woman 60/40 indica dom cross 16 to 18%THC (possible descendant of Ice) 2 phenotypes. One indica, like, the other sativa like. Habit of growth is classic indica with massive, tight flowers that are VERY sticky with trichomes. Vulnerable to mold does not do well in high humidity climates – best in Mediterranean climate …i.e. California. Produces impressively high yields.

Good For: Muscle Spasms, Fatigue, Stress, Sexual Arousal, Pain, Insomnia

Possible Side Effects: Euphoria, Paranoia – less frequently reported: Dry Mouth, Dry Eyes, occasionally Headache

Black Haze 60/40 sativa dom cross   22%THC (Colombian Black x Columbian Gold x Purple Haze) Known for its very dark purple buds – so dark they appear black - hence the name. (Beware: there are autoflowering strains with entirely different parentage going by this name. While they may have virtues of their own, they are not the strain of which we are speaking) Tastes woody, earthy with a slight hint of sweet berry.

No horticultural info available.

Good For: Sexual Arousal, Pain, Stress, Depression, Seizures, Migraines

Possible Side Effects: Relaxed even if active, Dry Eyes, Dry Mouth, with only a tiny minority of patients reporting Dry Eyes and an even smaller number a tinge of Dizziness, Headache and/or Paranoia

K-Train 85/15 indica dominant cross to 23%THC (OG Kush x Trainwreck) by Greenhouse Seeds. Easy to grow indoors or out. Yields 900g /m² indoors, 1,000g/plant outdoors. Flowering time of 9 weeks

Good For: Sexual Arousal, Relaxation. Depression, Pain

Possible Side Effects: Relaxed, Happy, Euphoric, Dry Mouth. Few reported Dry Eyes, and very few reported Dizziness, Paranoia and/or headache

Blue Zombie 70/30 indica dom cross 20 to 21%THC (Zombi OG x Unk. strain) Smells like fresh ground coffee, fuel, and skunky grape, with a similar taste. While there is grow info. on Zombie OG and Zombie Kush, there is none for Blue Zombie. Since it is a cross with an Unk. parent one would have to look at the habit of growth for Zombie OG and extrapolate possibilities from there.

Good For: Excellent for Pain/Chronic Pain, Insomnia, Appetite, Sexual Arousal, Muscle Spasms

Possible Side Effects: Euphoria, Creeper, Dry Mouth, Dry Eyes

Tropicali (AKA **Tropicali Kush**)

65/35 sativa dom cross   15 to 19%THC
breeder secrecy = Unk. parentage. Buds are dense,
popcorn shaped, covered in orange hairs and dense,
sticky trychomes.

Good For: Sexual Arousal, Stress, Depression,
Headache, Glaucoma, ADD/ADHD, Giggles

Possible Side Effects: Euphoric, Dry Mouth, some
Paranoia reported, fewer reports or Dry Eyes and very
few Headache

Orange Velvet indica dominant cross 18 to 22%THC
(Orange Skunk x Unknown) Said to have come from "an
old Hippie who had been growing it in the N.W. for 20
years," The smell, both in growing and smoking is said
to be unbelievable – just like oranges. One of the
parents of both Agent Orange and of Jillybean. Lacks
bag appeal, so is rarely commercially available but is
said to way make up for it in taste (also orange like).
No information on horticultural particulars available
but it is said to be well worth growing.

Good For: Sexual Arousal, Stress, Headaches,
Migraines, Eye Pressure, Appetite

Possible Side Effects: Euphoria, Relaxation, Dry
Mouth, some experience Anxiety, few experience
Dry Eyes, Paranoia and/or dizziness. Hard to find.

Purple Paralysis (AKA **Jellyfish Bud**)

sativa dominant cross   22%THC
(Power Plant x Lavender) by Cream of the Crop. This plant is resistant to both mold and bugs, has purple-blue flowers and grows both indoors and outdoors. Yield is 450g /m² indoors and 650g/plant outdoors. Flowers 9 to 10 weeks
Good For: Sexual Arousal, Stress, Relaxation, Pain

Possible Side Effects: Happy, Euphoric VERY Powerful.

Ken's Kush cross by   18 to 20%THC

(Granddaddy Purple x OG Kush x Sour Diesel) by Ken Estes. Can be grown indoors (or outside in warm climates only). Taste is a cross of berries, skunk and earthy grass. Grows medium to tall. Flowering Time is 11 to 13 weeks. Yield is "medium."
Good For: Stress, Relaxation, Sexual Arousal, Pain
Possible Side Effects: Happiness – others not reported

Sour Strawberry Diesel cross   to 28% THC

(Sour Strawberry x Turbo Diesel) by MTG Seeds. Chunky red and purple buds. Other source: (Sour Diesel x Strawberry Cough) 4% CBD // another source, (NTC Diesel x Strawberry Cough). Flowerins for 9 to 10 weeks. Yield unreported
Good For: Sexual Arousal, Stress

Possible Side Effects: Happy, Talkative, Anxiety, some Dizziness

Tangerine Man sativa dominant cross   18% THC
From Leafs by Snoop. One of Snoop Dog's favorite strains, Buds more dense than most sativas. No further horticultural information is available.
Good For: Stress, Fatigue, Sexual Arousal, Depression
Possible Side Effects: Good with physical activity, Happy, Euphoria, Anxiety

Hawaiian Delight 50/50 cross indica dom 20%THC
Most sources say little is known of this strain's origins but one source stated it was a cross of (Afghan x Skunk x Hawaiian Landrace) Aroma is musky hash like. Tastes on an earthy hash flavor. No information on growing this strain can be found.
Good For: Stress, Relaxation, Pain, Nausea, Depression, Fatigue, Sexual Arousal
Possible Side Effects: Happy, Dry Mouth. A minority reported Dizziness, Dry Eyes, Headache or Paranoia

Hell's Angel OG (AKA **Biker's Kush** and **Hell's OG**)
 80/20 indica dominant cross   20 to 24%THC
(OG Kush x Blackberry) NOTE: There is some debate on the parentage, origin, etc. Said to have been bred by the bikers themselves in Southern California. Other sources claim they took the strain and rights and the name from a breeder who "owed" them. (The first time

I smoked was with a group of Oakland Hells Angels in the summer of 1965. While they were congenial, they were definitely NOT people you would want to refuse if they felt you owed them. So,the latter story is quite believable to me.) Stories and myths abound, but the effects are agreed upon...Flowers for 8 to 9 weeks. (Another source says 9 to 11 weeks, but that seems unlikely due to the 80% Indica DNA)

Good For: PTSD, Pain, Stress, Depression, Relaxation, possible Sexual Arousal

Possible Side Effects: Comes on strong, NOT for beginners due to possibility of Paranoia and even hallucinations. Euphoria, Anxiety, Dry Eyes, Dry Mouth, Some Dizziness and/or Headache

Gumbo   65/35 indica dom cross   20%THC

Named after bubblegum, not the Cajun dish. Unknown origin or parentage. Plants are covered with trichome frost. The taste is intense, sweet and hashy with sugary bubble gum traces. Moderately difficult to grow. Flowers for 8 weeks. Yield is "medium." However, people love the taste and smell (considered one of the best 3 strains in terms of aroma) and it is quite good medicinally.

Good For: Muscular Dystrophy, Insomnia, Relaxation, Pain, Stress, Bipolar Disorder, Migraine, Glaucoma, may cause Sexual Arousal.

Possible Side Effects: Dry Mouth, some report Dry Eyes, few reported Headache very few Dizziness and/or Paranoia. Couchlock is likely

Honey Boo Boo 80/20indica dom cross 15 to 21%THC (Bubba Kush x Captain Krypt OG) by DNA Genetics Plant turns purple upon flowering, sweet, pleasing taste. Flowering period is 8 to 9 weeks. Yields 400 to 500g/m²

Good For: Sexual Arousal, Relaxation, insomnia, Stress, Pain

Possible Side Effects: Happiness, Anxiety

Thai Haze 80/20 sative dominant cross   21%THC (Thai X Haze) Grows over six feet, difficult to grow, exceptionally long flowering period of 14 to 16 weeks. Plants to 7 feet tall, not easily grown/not beginner grow

Good For: Depression, Stress, Sexual Arousal

Possible Side Effects: Comes on slowly then becomes intense. Experienced users who like haze are pleased. Anxiety potential high, some reported headache.

Serious 6 almost pure sativa cross   17%THC (Canadian land race sativas x African landrace sativas) by Serious Seeds. Easily grown outdoors but only recommended for expert growers indoors. It is a vigorous grower. Flowering time is only 8 weeks. Yield is 350 to 500g/m²

Good For: Stress, Creativity, Energy, Depression, Sexual Arousal

Possible Side Effects: Happiness, Anxiety many have Dry Eyes, Dry Mouth

Twista 50/50 cross, sativa dominant 19+%THC
(Shiva x Trainwreck) 3rd place 2014 Denver Cannabis
Cup. Though balanced, it has both a sativa effect and
habit of growth. Produces long buds. Described as
"Smooth." Further growing information unavailable.
Good For: Sexual Arousal, Creativity, Depression,
Stress
Possible Side Effects: Uplifting, Dry Mouth, Anxiety all
highly reported.

Killing Fields sativa dominant cross   22%THC
(The One x Jack) by Sannie's Seeds. Plant grows tall.
Has green/blue buds. Strong fruity odor. Several
phenotypes. Flowers for 11-13 weeks. Yield is
"Medium."
Good For: Sexual Arousal, Stress, Depression,
Creativity, Fatigue
Possible Side Effects: "Up," Dry Mouth, many
patients report Dry Eyes, Headache while a
considerable number report Dizziness and/or
Paranoia.

Santa Maria F8 75/25 sativa dom cross12 to14%THC
(Santa Maria x Mexican Haze x Silver Pearl, then back-
crossed four generations). by No Mercy Seeds A male
from that generation was then bred with a pure Santa
Maria mother, which was then inbred 8 times) – possibly
the most complex breeding program of any strain.
Grows best outside under natural light. However, even
outdoors it requires pruning or it keeps growing and

will eventually break from the weight of its flowers. Staking is an absolute must. Cut for vertical growth will result in a bushier plant that can hold itself better. Flowering is 8 to 9 weeks. Yield is said to be "very high" but no figures are available.

Good For: Erotic response, Stress, Depression,

Possible Side Effects: Sexual Response is limited to the F8 phenotype of Santa Maria, choose your seed company carefully. Dry Eyes, Dizziness, Anxiety are all frequently reported

CBD Yummy (AKA **Yummy)70/30 sativa dom cross 1:1 CBD:THC (average) 5%CBD (average): 5%THC (Granddaddy Kush x White Dawg) by CBD Crew Large Colas, strong plant. Flowers for 8 to 9 weeks. Yield is 400g/m^2 indoors

Good For: Stress, Pain, Depression, Inflammation, Insomnia. Pos Sexual Arousal

Possible Side Effects: Anxiety. Some patients reported Arousal. A very popular strain with relatively short lived effects.

Lemon Kush Indica   21%THC
(Master Kush x Lemon Joy) There are at least 2 phenotypes of Lemon Kush and more than one breed lines. Some consider one far superior to the other.... (one of the phenotypes of the above listed parentage). The best of all the Kush crosses. Does best in organic grow. Flowers for 8 to 9 weeks, Yields are referred to as "average."

Good For: Uplifting, Stress, Depression, Pain,

sometimes Erotic.

Possible Side Effects: Very strong, Euphoria, Dry Mouth, Dry Eyes, few report Anxiety, Paranoia and/or Dizziness.

Brooklyn Mango 50/50 cross   14 to 21%THC
(Ed Rosenthal Super Bud x NYC Diesel) by Dr. Underground. Smells like tangy mango with sweet earthiness. Tastes like a mix of pineapple, mango and lemon with a diesel flavor upon exhale. Grows well indoors/outdoors. Flowers 8 to 9 weeks. Yield indoors using SOG or SCROG is 500 to 700g/m^2 Outdoors 800 to 1,000g/plant or more.

Good For: Tinnitus, Sexual Arousal, Stress, Depression Inspiration, Creativity.

Possible Side Effects: NOTE: high levels of reported Anxiety, Dry Eyes, Dry Mouth, Dizziness NOT recommended for beginners or patients with Anxiety

Cherry Cola (NOT Cherry Kola)
                    indica dom cross   %THC Unk.
Very little can be found on this strain

Good For: Sexual Arousal, Stress, Pain, Depression

Possible Side Effects: NOTE: Due to frequency of negative side effects this medication is not recommended for any but those highly experienced in handling said effects: Anxiety, Dizziness, Dry Mouth and Paranoia were all reported at high levels.

Growing Hints

SOIL: Personally, I am 100% organic on everything I grow, however, I am aware everyone may not be....pity. It is easy to find an abundance of organic fertilizer for the grow stage of the plants. It is most important the percentage of compost you use in mixing your soil is HIGH. If you have access to local compost, use it! Do a little reading and include lots of compost, bedding soil and for water retention (and cost efficiency) I like pressed coconut husk that swells up when exposed to moisture. It is also worth noting that you do NOT have to throw away soil after one year. You DO have to mix it with about equal amounts of compost, new soil and worm castings and be conscientious re fertilizing

FERTILIZATION: For fertilization, basically, you want a similar regimen as for tomatoes BUT at about ½ the level. You want trace minerals and a good amount of nitrogen rich fertilizer, such as fish fertilizer. REMEMBER, use about half what the directions say! When the plants begin to flower you need to STOP using nitrogen. To increasing bloom numbers and size it is important when you plants first start to bloom to use a fertilizer high in potassium and very low to zero Nitrogen. I use Langbeinite (0-0-22) with an exceptionally high level of potassium (just what you want for an organic bloom booster. Fish bone is also good – but not as good – and very inexpensive. For more information search Youtube, especially Jeorge Cervantes as well as his Cannabis Encyclopedia. The ultimate guide is Encyclopedia of Organic Gardening Hardcover, 1978. You can get it used for a few dollars. (the one attributed to the editors of Organic Gardening is fine as well., but I like the older one . Get terrific book prices by searching: http://used.addall.com

CONTAINERS: Besides for your soil mix and fertilization, crucial
to your yield will be the diameter of your planter. Most single home
growers plant either indoors or outdoors use 15 gal. planters commonly found in any nursery supply. However, it is the diameter that really matters most. Cannabis does not have a tap root. It is a wide-root grower. a 4 or 5 ft. diameter planter 18" to 2 Ft. deep is capable of growing a MONSTER sized plant (the plant roots will only use the top 16' to 18"). I mean with a trunk as big as the thick part of a baseball bat and dozens and dozens of colas. Various sized planting canvas bags are available form "Hydroponic" grow shops and can also be found on line. If at all possible, do not get black planters, as the sun will burn the roots when they reach the edge (and they will reach the edge). With few exceptions, harvest when 70% the trichomes have turned opaque and about 30% are already or are becoming amber in color. That is the ultimate harvest time for nearly all strains. Past 30% amber and the THC levels drop and the flower is past optimum potency. There should be no clear trichomes at harvest time. A simple 10 X jeweler's loop is perfect for close examination of the trichomes. For best results one must never harvest early or late. For a few particular strains other percentages apply. You've gone to all the trouble and you want optimum yield and potency. With some strains listed you will harvest top colas first and lower ones later WATER: If you live in a "hard water" area you need to use an in-line   filter.   I   use   two   in   line.   A   great

option is a large child's wading pool (up to about 3 Ft. x 8 Ft. at Wallmart or other source. Grow some plants (Water Lilies, Carnivorous plants, etc. and BE SURE to have mosquito fish. Avery inexpensive water pump can be had to run a $10 head that can later be used to switch over to a hose when you are ready to water. Then fill the pool up and let it aerate via the fountain until the

next watering. Whenever possible, water with compost "tea." (Look   it   up)

Recommended Organic Insecticide, Caterpillar and Disease Control Mix

Throughout the course of cannabis growth the plants are susceptible to various insects and diseases. One that particularly frustrates me is the caterpillar of a particular butterfly that hatches in the bloom and kills all the bloom above where it is happily munching away. Indoor growers are subject to spider mites even more than outdoor growers and they can destroy the entire grow room in a couple of days! Personally, I am totally into organic fertilizing as well as spray, (however, I accept that many are not so inclined and will utilize other fertilizing regimens). Regardless, the one arena in which organics is a "NO BRAINER" is insect and disease control. There is a simple, method of organically controlling these problems that is unsurpassed in efficiency and is cheaper than the use of toxic poison on your plants! It is a combination listed below that will control Mold, Rust, Mildew, and every critter including caterpillars and the truly difficult Spider Mite! ALL ingredients are available through Amazon and are very reasonably priced:

Dr. Bronner's Fair Trade and Organic Sal Suds Liquid Cleaner

SaferGro Mildew Cure, Organic Fungicide

Super Clean Neem Oil

RiD Bugs Organic Insecticide

Thuricide (Bacillus thuringensis) 8 oz.
Mix the above in a quart sized container in warm water, then add to the water in your sprayer.

The above combination will do everything you need to keep your plants safe as well as yourself. If you have only 3 to 6 plants, less than one quart of the above spray is all you will need per use. If you have any doubts as to frequency, and definitely when blooming has begun, spray every 4 days. It is a bit of a pain in the ass, but is safe and MUCH less difficult than dealing with the loss of your harvest. If, like me, you have a large vegetable garden and/or other plants, 1 gallon is best. Regardless, the above items will last you several seasons. If you only have a few plants, you can get a 1-gallon sprayer for under $20. However, THE ne plus ultra is a professional fogger, which assures total coverage, is a one-time investment and can be had from Amazon as per below:

Hudson 99598 Fog Electric Atomizer Sprayer, Commercial/portable: $195.19

If you use the sprayer and not the fogger, be sure to saturate the underside of your plants as well as the surface. NOTE: I just discovered my grow store now has a small hand sprayer that builds up pressure and emits an exceptionally fine mist. For an individual with only one to three plants this might be the ideal compromise re coverage and cost.

Glossary

Autoflowering Strains that flower automatically, regardless of light changes, typically 30 to 90 days (depending on the strain) due to influx of Cannabis rudaralis genes in their parental background. "Normal" strains flower for various periods depending on the strain but flowering onset occurs due to a change in number of hours of light in the day – hence, "harvest time." Autoflowering strains take on the automatic flowering cycle of the C. rudaralis resulting in a crop which varies by strain from about 30 daysto 75 days from seed to harvest depending on the strain. This allows for multiple harvests during the planting season, but they are of course, smaller plants – which can be very desirable for indoor grows.

Cannabinoids (CBD and THC are the most talked about) are the chemical compounds secreted by cannabis plants, with the highest concentration bing in the flowers – or "buds"). They provide relief to an array of symptoms as well as maintaining internal stability and health. Cannabis contains at least 85 types of cannabinoids, many of which have documented medical value.

Clone Common term for an individual plant grown from taking a cutting from a "mother" plant and rooting it. It will have the same genetic make up as the "parent" plant. Hence the term, "clone," but in fact, the proper

32

horticultural term is a "cutting." (A true clone comes from a far more complex process – however, the result is the same – a plant identical in genetics to the "parent" plant)

Cola (AKA **Kola**) A bloom stalk.

Couch-lock Completely free of movement for extended periods of time. Usually accompanied by profound relaxation.

Cotton mouth "Dry mouth." Lacking in normal saliva flow. A common side effect of many strains of cannabis.

Charas (AKA **Finger Hash**) A psychoactive concentrate made by hand-rubbing live mature female cannabis flowers to collect the resin. It is the oldest form of concentrate as well at the simplest and most efficient method to collect fresh resin from cannabis plants. Best done at the peak of their flowering cycle.

Creeper A strain that seems to have little effect initially, but after a period of time (5 to 20 minutes) comes to full effect – with some strains the full effect gradually grows and grows while with other strains following the delay it can manifest suddenly.

D.W.C. (Deep Water Culture) A hydroponic system – beyond the scope of this work – easily researched on the net and available via Amazon as well as any hydroponics store.

Entourage Effect Dynamics whereby cannabis compounds that have minimal or no effect in isolation may generate significant effects when combined with additional cannabinoids and terpenes. Put simply, the beneficial impact of the whole plant is greater than the sum of its individual parts (cannabinoids).

F1, F2, etc. F1 refers to the resulting plants from a cross. However, F2 refers to the plants resulting from crossing two F1s. F3, from crossing two F2s, etc. This is continued until a desired trait or traits are "stabilized" and can be expected in the vast majority of resulting seeds.

Finger Hash (AKA **Charas**) A psychoactive concentrate made by hand-rubbing live mature female cannabis flowers to collect the resin. It is the oldest form of concentrate as well at the simplest and most efficient method to collect fresh resin from cannabis plants. Best done at the peak of their flowering cycle.

Genotype The entire genetic heritage of an individual plant or animal (carried in the DNA of each and every cell of same individual)

Hydroponics A system of growing plants in a foam type medium submerged

IBL Inbred line. Bred back to itself repeatedly. This is done to at least the 4th generation (F4) to stabilize a given trait or traits to assure they will appear in vast majority of plants from seed.

Kola (AKA **Cola**) A bloom stalk.

Lollipopping is a pruning technique whereby one prunes off the lower branches, hence giving a lollipop appearance to the plant. Thisallows for free air flow (which reduces disease incidence) and the energy of the plant to be put into the larger branches that will,therefore produce larger flowers.

m² Square meter – a bit larger than a square yard- 39 x 39" – a common method of reporting the number of grams an indoor grow will yield. Indoor grows are typically reported in this manor while outdoor grows are typically reported as grams per plant. Both reference the resulting trimmed and cured (semi-dried) buds (flowers) produced.

Marijuana The common name for the genus cannabis – primarily used in reference to cannabis sativa and cannabis indica, the two species that create an altered state of consciousness when ingested. (derived from the early use in the U.S. almost always imported then from

Mexico where the slang name was "Mary Jane {Eng.} – Marijuana {Spanish}")

Munchies Profound desire to eat – sometimes odd combinations of food.

OG The origin of this title in a strain's name is wildly debated with no less than 4 separate claims as to its origin. 1) Many say it stands for **"**Ocean Grown," denoting strains developed along the Northern California coastal areas were temperatures are moderate, there is plenty of sunlight, moisture from fog and relatively frequent rain. 2) However, the developer and namesake for all the "Kush" strains is a fellow named, O.G. Kush, so that would account for all the original strains

35

containing OG in their name. 3) Yet another claim is that it stands for Organically Grown. 4) The final theoretical origin is the idea that it stands for "Original Gangster" – meaning a gangster that has been around for some time, thereby "righteous," dependable and worthy of respect. Additionally, I have heard that some breeders who now attach "OG" to any strain they consider exceptional, regardless of origin.

Phenotype Individual physical manifestations within a given strain. Like people, each plant individually grown from seed is unique. This variation occurs only among individual plants grown from seed but not among clones (cuttings) of a specific Individual, all of which have identical genetic make up. When a breeder cross pollinates strains and then plants the seeds s/he will end up with hundreds of differing phenotypes. Usually the one with the very best traits will be the only one from which cuttings are taken ("clones") and which receives a new name. However, sometimes there are two or more phenotypes which are given different or the same name – fortunately, this is relatively rare.

SCROG Screen of Green – utilizing a netting system to produce a "carpet" or "Sea" of green tops which tend to all mature into flowering at the same time – commonly used in indoor artificial lighting environments and believed to produce the highest yield.

Sinsemilla (literally, Spanish for "without seeds) grown with the male plants removed from the area the females are grown, hence preventing fertilization of the flowers and allowing the plant to spend more energy producing larger flowers, higher THC levels rather than expend that energy developing seeds.

SOG "Sea Of Green" – a growing method where all the branches of all plants are cut to the same height to produce a "carpet" or "Sea" of green tops which tend to all mature into flowering at the same time – commonly used in indoor artificial lighting environments and believed to produce the highest yield. When netting is used to achieve this it is referred to as SCROG, or Screen of Green. (See above).

Smooth This refers to the easy smoking characteristic of some strains that do not cause coughing or the like. Easy to take.

Super Cropping A method to increase the number of "tops" of a cannabis plant in order to push the lower growth higher and wider so that all the branches will flower. It involves semi-breaking the tallest growth and bending it at a right angle, rather than pruning it off. See reports via google and You Tube. Many growers swear it, "...allows the nutrients to work double duty, producing much heavier yields in areas that wouldn't have been particularly productive. The plants themselves tend to look bushier and more robust as a result of super cropping."

Terpenes Elements in marijuana that increase dopamine activity (as in "runners' high"), effect the smell and the flavor of a given strain as well as activate neurotransmitters and receptors.

THC (Tetrahydrocannabinal) The cannabinoid causing mind altering effects found in highest concentration in the flowers of the female cannabis plant. It is also in very high concentrations in the small leaves in the flower cola (though commercially this is inanely trimmed away). Also, to a much lower degree it is found in the leaves of the female plant. It is not found in the leaves of the male plant nor in male or female Cannabis ruderalus.

THCV (Tetrahydrocannabivarin) This is a cannabinoid that paradoxically inhibits appetite when reaching 1% or higher. This is rare among strains as most strains increase appetite and some cause one to be ravenous.

Top Shelf This is primarily a marketing term meant to get top dollar for either strains with very high THC count (i.e. 20% and up) or strains that carry particularly good reputations.

Trichomes The small resin glands present on the flowers and main small leaves of the bloom in late-stage cannabis plants. This is where the THC, CBD and other medical properties are located. The development of the trichomes is the main indicator of time to harvest. However, there are several variations depending on the desired outcome. For the clearest mental effects, one wants to harvest as the trichomes have turned opaque and about 10% are turning amber. The time from from when they begin to "turn amber" to the point they are 50%+ amber is only a day or two, so, a plant must be closely observed (with a jeweler's loupe) to know when exactly to harvest. BTW, many commercial growers wait until the 50%+ amber stage as a matter of course, as that is when the buds will be reaching maximum weight.

Bibliography
Books & Articles:

Americans for Safe Access, *Multiple Sclerosis and Medical Cannabis An ASA Guide* Published by Americans for Safe Access Foundation 2013 Kindle Edition.

Backes, Michael: *Cannabis Pharmacy The Practical Guide*
to Medical Marijuana, Elephant Book Company, Ltd. 2014

Barcott, Bruce & Scherer, Michael: "The Highly Divisive, Curiously

Underfunded and Strangely Promising World of Pot Science"
Time Magazine, May 25, 2015

Bello, Joan: *The Benefits Of Marijuana: Physical, Psychological and Spiritual*, Lifeservices Press, Susquehanna, Pennsylvania, 2008

Conrad, Chris, *Hemp For Health: The Medicinal and Nutritional Uses of Cannabis Sativa*, Healing Arts Press, Rochester, Vermont, 1997

Danko, Danny, *25 Years Of Growing Chem Dog*, High Times, October, 2016

Danko, Danny, *The Official HIGH TIMES Field Guide to Marijuana Strains*
High Times Books, New York, NY 2010,

Des Barres, Xander, *2014 Cannabis Guide to the Best Strains*,

Eternal Bhodi Books. Los Angeles, California, 2013

J.I. Rodale, 1978 *Encyclopedia of Organic Gardening*, (Hardcover), Rodale Press, Emmaus, PA, 1978

Grinspoon, Lester MD. "Marijuana and the Forbidden Medicine" 1997

J.I. Rodale, 1978 *Encyclopedia of Organic Gardening*, Rodale Press, (Hardcover)

J, Sirius, "Highest THCV Strains," High Times, January 29, 2015

Lee, Martin A. *Smoke Signals: A Social History of Marijuana—Medical, Recreational and Scientific*, Scribner Publishing, NY, NY 2012

McGill, Jenna, *Cannabis: Complete Guide to Medicinal Marijuana as a Holistic Medicine – Medicinal Usage and Health Benefits of Cannabis*, Medical Marijuana for Health, ... Healing, and Alternative

Medicine Book 2). JMW Publishing Company. Kindle Edition.

Oner, S. T, *Cannabis indica: The Essential Guide To The World's Finest Marijuana Strains Vol. 1*, Green Candy Press, San Francisco, California 2011

Oner, S. T, *Cannabis indica: The Essential Guide To The World's Finest Marijuana Strains Vol. 2*, Green Candy Press, San Francisco, California 2013

Oner, S. T, *Cannabis indica: The Essential Guide To The World's Finest Marijuana Strains Vol. 3*, Green Candy Press, San Francisco, California 2013

Oner, S. T, *Cannabis sativa: The Essential Guide To The World's Finest Marijuana Strains Vol. 1*, Green Candy Press, San Francisco, California 2012

Oner, S. T, *Cannabis sativa: The Essential Guide To The World's Finest Marijuana Strains Vol. 2*, Green Candy Press, San Francisco, California 2013

Oner, S. T, *Cannabis sativa: The Essential Guide To The*

World's Finest Marijuana Strains Vol. 3, Green Candy
Press, San Francisco, California 2014

Pabon, Richard, *Marijuana and Sex*
Kindle Edition

Pabon, Richard, *Marijuana and Autism*
Kindle Edition, 2014

Potter,Dr. Beverly and Joy, Dan, *The Healing Magic of
Cannabis*, Ronin Publishing, Berkeley, California, 1998

Saint Thomans, Sophe, "The Stoner Orgasmm," High
Times,
January, 2016

Werner, Clint, *Marijuana: Gateway to Health*, Dachstar
Press, San Francisco, California, 2011

"Miss September: Meizy Chiang," High Times,
September, 2015

Online sources:

Annunaki Genetics
http://www.annunakigenetics.com

420 Magazine
http://www.420magazine.com

420 Resources
http://www.420resource.net

All Bud
https://www.allbud.com

Blog
http://blog.sfgate.com

Boards Cannabis
http://boards.cannabis.com

Brothers Grimm Seeds
http://www.brothersgrimmseeds.com

Buds Guru
https://budsguru.com

Buds and Roses (Carry Joy's Strain, inc. Oil)
http://www.budsandrosesla.com

Bud Tender
https://ibudtender.com

Bud Vibes
https://www.budvibes.com

Cannabis Now Magazine
http://cannabisnowmagazine.com

Cannabis Pocket Reference
http://degausspress.com

Canna Info
https://cannafo.com

Cannasos.com
https://cannasos.com

CBD Crew
http://cbdcrew.org

Clone Queen Genetics
http://www.cqdna.com

Culture Magazine
http://ireadculture.com

Dark Heart Nursary
http://darkheartnursery.com

Devil's Harvest Seeds
https://thedevilsharvestseeds.com

DNA Genetics
http://dnagenetics.com

Dutch Seeds
https://www.buydutchseeds.com

EN Seedfinder
http://en.seedfinder.eu

Evolab
http://www.evolab.com

Gorilla Glue Strains
http://www.gorillaglue4.com

Grow 4 Me
http://gro4me.com

Grow Marijuana.com
http://grow-marijuana.com

Harborside Health Center
https://www.harborsidehealthcenter.com

Herbal Dispatch
http://herbaldispatch.com

Herbies Headshop
http://www.herbiesheadshop.com

High Times (on line)
http://hightimes.com/grow/the-best-cbd-strains-of-2015/

How To Grow Marijuanna
http://howtogrowmarijuana.com

How to Grow Weed 420
http://howtogrowweed420.com

Hmblt Delivery Devices
http://hmbldt.com/delivery-devices/

International Cannagraphic
https://www.icmag.com

Kind Green Buds
http://www.kindgreenbuds.com

Kyle Kushman
http://kylekushman.com

Ladybud
https://www.ladybud.com/2015/02/02/joeys-strain-cannabis-created-for-symptoms-related-to-autism/

Leafy
www.leafly.com

Marijuana.com
http://www.marijuana.com

Marijuana Doctors
https://www.marijuanadoctors.com

Marijuana Growing
http://www.marijuanagrowing.com

Marijuana Seed Strain Review.com
http://www.marijuanaseedstrainreview.com

Mary's Nutritionals
http://www.marysnutritionals.com/category-s/102.htm

MedicalJane
http://www.medicaljane.com

medicalmerijuanastrains.com

http://www.medicalmarijuanastrains.com/strain-guide/

Medireview.com
http://medireview.com

Michigan Medical Marijuana Association
http://michiganmedicalmarijuana.org

NARCONON
http://www.narconon.org/drug-information/marijuana-history.html

National Academies of Sciences, *The Health Effects of*

Cannabis and Cannabinoids,
https://www.nap.edu/catalog/24625/the-health-
effects-of-cannabis-and-cannabinoids-the-current-state

News THC
https://www.newsthc.com

Original Sensible Seeds
http://original-ssc.com

Pot Guide
https://potguide.com

Porter, Nanette, *Canabus Plant Anatomy: Trichomes 101,*
Medical Jane, on-line
https://www.medicaljane.com/2017/03/11/trichomes/

Project CBD
https://www.projectcbd.org

The Cannabist
http://www.thecannabist.co

The Nug
http://www.thenug.com

The WeedBlog
http://www.theweedblog.com

Original Sensible Seed Company
http://original-ssc.com

Project CBD
https://www.projectcbd.org

Project CBD
https://www.projectcbd.org/?utm_source=ZohoCampai

gns&utm_campaign=Project+CBD+Newsfeed+%2807-19-2016%29_2016-07-18_1&utm_medium=email

Rhino Seeds
http://www.cannabis-seeds.co.uk

Rough, Lisa, *Do Cannabis-Infused Suppositories Actually Work? We Tried One to Find Out*, Leafly, www.leafly.com 2017

Royal Queen Seed
http://www.royalqueenseeds.com

Science Daily
https://www.sciencedaily.com

Seed Finder
http://en.seedfinder.eu

Southern Humbold Seed Collective
https://www.kingofcbdgenetics.com/sohum-seed-genetics

Spirit Smoker
http://spiritsmoker.tumblr.com

Stickyguide
http://91life.stickyguide.com

Strain Brain
http://www.strainbrain.com

Swamies Medical Marijuana Dispensary
https://swamis420.wordpress.com

THC Finder
http://www.thcfinder.com

The Cannabist Company
http://www.thecannabist.co

The Weed Blog
http://www.theweedblog.com

True Herbal Care
http://www.trueherbalcare.com

Weed Yard
http://weedyard.com

Wikileaf
http://www.wikileaf.com

Dear Reader,

I would like to personally thank you for ordering this book and invite you to leave a brief review on the site of purchase. Don't keep this information a secret.

Please mention in your review what drew you to the book, if the book delivered on what the title promised, if your impression is that the book is of value to current or prospective medical marijuana patients and/or to patients considering which strains they may want to consider for growing and any other comments you deem relevant. Any author loves seeing five star reviews, but I assure you ANY HONEST REVIEW will be highly valued, appreciated and I thank you in advance.
Sincerely,

Michael Blood, Author